IMG Friendly Transitional Year Residency
Programs List

With Comprehensive Match Selection Criteria
and Programs Requirements

By

IMG Guide

And

Applicant Guide

Introduction

IMG Friendly Transitional Year Residency Programs

In Collaboration between the Applicant Guide and the IMG Guide we present to you the most complete and up-to-date IMG friendly transitional year residency programs list with full match selection criteria and requirements for these programs. This book is essentially written for international medical graduates seeking residency in the US. The idea of writing this book came from our insight that many IMGs every year don't match because they don't know where to apply. Most of the time, they end applying to programs that don't have IMGs or those that don't match their criteria hence they end losing money with no interviews earned. The information was gathered from program directors, coordinators, chiefs, faculty and residents. It includes Programs names, Programs codes, States, Addresses, Phones, Faxes, Percentage of IMGs in the programs, Minimum USMLE Step 1 and Step 2 Score Requirements, Attempts on any step, CS requirement at time of application, USCE Requirements, Cut-Off time since graduation, Programs offering couple match and Visas Sponsored or accepted.

Connecticut

Yale-New Haven Hospital Transitional Year Residency Program

Specialty: Transitional Year
Program name: Yale-New Haven Hospital Program
Program code: 999-08-00-020
NRMP Code: 1090999P0
Program type: University-based
State: Connecticut

Address: Yale New Haven, Transitional Year
Program
　　　　1450 Chapel St, New Haven, CT
06511-4440
Phone: (203) 789-3989
Fax: (203) 789-3222
Percentage of IMGs in the program: 30%
Minimum USMLE Step 1 Score Requirement:
No limits set
Minimum USMLE Step 2 Score Requirement:
No limits set
Attempts on any step: Must pass on first
attempt
CS required at time of application: Yes
USCE Requirement: None
Cut-Off time since graduation: 3 years
Program offers couple match: Yes
Visas Sponsored or accepted: J1 visa

St. Vincent Medical Center Transitional Year Residency Program

Specialty: Transitional Year
Program name: St Vincent's Medical Center
Program
Program code: 999-08-00-018
NRMP Code: 1080999P0

Program type: Community-based university affiliated hospital
State: Connecticut
Address: St Vincent's Medical Center, Transitional Year Program,
2800 Main St, Bridgeport, CT 06606
Phone: 203 576 5578

Percentage of IMGs in the program: 80%
Minimum USMLE Step 1 Score Requirement: 210
Minimum USMLE Step 2 Score Requirement: 210
Attempts on any step: No limits set
CS required at time of application: Yes
USCE Requirement: None
Cut-Off time since graduation: 10 years
Program offers couple match: Yes
Visas Sponsored or accepted: J1 visa and H1b visa

Georgia

The Medical Center Transitional Year Residency Program

Specialty: Transitional Year
Program name: The Medical Center Program
Program code: 999-12-00-229
NRMP Code: 1118999P0
Program type: Community-based
State: Georgia
Address: The Medical Center Inc, Suite 100
          1900 10th Ave, Columbus, GA
31902
Phone: (706) 571-1430
Fax: (706) 571-1604
Percentage of IMGs in the program: 20%
Minimum USMLE Step 1 Score Requirement: No limits set
Minimum USMLE Step 2 Score Requirement: No limits set
Attempts on any step: No limits set
CS required at time of application: Yes
USCE Requirement: None
Cut-Off time since graduation: 5 years
Program offers couple match: Yes
Visas Sponsored or accepted: No

Emory University Transitional Year Residency Program

Specialty: Transitional Year
Program name: Emory University Program
Program code: 999-12-00-026
Program type: University-based
State: Georgia
Address: Grady Memorial Hospital,
           49 Jesse Hill Jr Dr SE, Atlanta, GA 30303
Phone: (404) 778-0263
Fax: (404) 778-1601
Percentage of IMGs in the program: 10%
Minimum USMLE Step 1 Score Requirement: 230
Minimum USMLE Step 2 Score Requirement: 230
Attempts on any step: Must pass on first attempt
CS required at time of application: Yes
USCE Requirement: None
Cut-Off time since graduation: 3 years
Program offers couple match: Yes
Visas Sponsored or accepted: J1 visa and H1b visa

Illinois

Swedish Covenant Hospital Transitional Year Residency Program

Specialty: Transitional Year
Program name: Swedish Covenant Hospital Program
Program code: 999-16-00-231
State: Illinois
Address: Swedish Covenant Hospital,
　　　5145 N California Avenue, Chicago, Illinois 60625
Phone: (773) 989-3808
Percentage of IMGs in the program: 20%
Minimum USMLE Step 1 Score Requirement: No limits set
Minimum USMLE Step 2 Score Requirement: No limits set
Attempts on any step: No limits set
CS required at time of application: No
USCE Requirement: None
Cut-Off time since graduation: No limits set
Program offers couple match: Yes
Visas Sponsored or accepted: No visa

Maryland

Maryland General Hospital Transitional Year Residency Program

Specialty: Transitional Year
Program name: University of Maryland Medical Center Midtown Campus Program
Program code: 999-23-00-049
State: Maryland
Address: Maryland General Hospital,
827 Linden Ave, Baltimore, MD 21201
Phone: (410) 225-8790
Fax: (410) 225-8910
Percentage of IMGs in the program: 80%
Minimum USMLE Step 1 Score Requirement: 205
Minimum USMLE Step 2 Score Requirement: 205
Attempts on any step: Must pass on first attempt
CS required at time of application: No
USCE Requirement: None
Cut-Off time since graduation: 5 years
Program offers couple match: No
Visas Sponsored or accepted: J1 visa

Harbor Hospital Center Transitional Year Residency Program

Specialty: Transitional Year
Program name: Harbor Hospital Center Program
Program code: 999-23-00-050
NRMP Code: 1250999P0
Program type: Community-based
State: Maryland
Address: MedStar Harbor Hospital, 3001 S Hanover St, Baltimore, MD 21225
Phone: (410) 350-3565
Fax: (410) 354-0186
Percentage of IMGs in the program: 50%
Minimum USMLE Step 1 Score Requirement: 230
Minimum USMLE Step 2 Score Requirement: 230
Attempts on any step: Must pass on first attempt
CS required at time of application: No
USCE Requirement: None
Cut-Off time since graduation: No limits set
Program offers couple match: Yes
Visas Sponsored or accepted: J1 visa

Massachusetts

MetroWest Medical Center/Harvard Medical School Transitional Year Residency Program

Specialty: Transitional Year
Program name: MetroWest Medical Center/Harvard Medical School Program
Program code: 999-24-00-160
NRMP Code: 1812999P0
Program type: Community-based university affiliated hospital
State: Massachusetts
Address: MetroWest Medical Center,
          115 Lincoln St, Framingham, MA 01702
Phone: (508) 383-1555
Fax: (508) 872-4794
Percentage of IMGs in the program: 50%
Minimum USMLE Step 1 Score Requirement: 205
Minimum USMLE Step 2 Score Requirement: 205
Attempts on any step: No limits set
CS required at time of application: No
USCE Requirement: None

Cut-Off time since graduation: 5 years unless clinically active as in residency or practice
Program offers couple match: Yes
Visas Sponsored or accepted: J1 visa

Michigan

Oakwood Heritage Hospital Transitional Year Residency Program

Specialty: Transitional Year
Program name: Oakwood Heritage Hospital Program
Program code: 999-25-00-258
Program type: Community-based university affiliated hospital
State: Michigan
Address: Oakwood Heritage Hospital,
          18101 Oakwood Blvd, Dearborn, MI 48124
Phone: (313) 436-2581
Fax: (313) 436-2071
Percentage of IMGs in the program: 15%
Minimum USMLE Step 1 Score Requirement: 210
Minimum USMLE Step 2 Score Requirement: 210

Attempts on any step: Must pass on first attempt
CS required at time of application: No
USCE Requirement: Yes
Cut-Off time since graduation: 5 years
Program offers couple match: No
Visas Sponsored or accepted: No visa

St. Mary Mercy Hospital Transitional Year Residency Program

Specialty: Transitional Year
Program name: St Mary Mercy Hospital Program
Program code: 999-25-00-255
NRMP Code: 1418999P0
Program type: Community-based
State: Michigan
Address: St Mary Mercy Hospital,
             36475 Five Mile Rd, Livonia, MI 48154
Phone: (734) 655-2704
Fax: (734) 655-8430
Percentage of IMGs in the program: 25%
Minimum USMLE Step 1 Score Requirement:
No limits set
Minimum USMLE Step 2 Score Requirement:
No limits set
Attempts on any step: Must pass on first attempt
CS required at time of application: No

USCE Requirement: None
Cut-Off time since graduation: 3 years
Program offers couple match: Yes
Visas Sponsored or accepted: J1 visa

Wayne State University School of Medicine Transitional Year Residency Program

Specialty: Transitional Year
Program name: Wayne State University School of Medicine Program
Program code: 999-25-00-253
NRMP Code: 1361999P0
Program type: University-based
State: Michigan
Address: Crittenton Hospital Medical Center,
          1101 W University Dr, Rochester, MI
48307
Phone: (248) 601-4900
Fax: (248) 601-4994
Percentage of IMGs in the program: 15%
Minimum USMLE Step 1 Score Requirement: 205
Minimum USMLE Step 2 Score Requirement: 205
Attempts on any step: Must pass on first attempt including CS exam
CS required at time of application: No
USCE Requirement: 6 months

Cut-Off time since graduation: 5 years
Program offers couple match: Yes
Visas Sponsored or accepted: J1 visa

Providence Hospital and Medical Centers Transitional Year Residency Program

Specialty: Transitional Year
Program name: Providence Hospital and Medical Centers Program
Program code: 999-25-00-068
NRMP Code: 1303999P1, 1303999P0
Program type: Community-based
State: Michigan
Address: Providence Hospital and Medical Center,
                16001 W Nine Mile Rd, Southfield, MI 48075
Phone: (248) 849-8441
Fax: (248) 849-5324
Percentage of IMGs in the program: 40%
Minimum USMLE Step 1 Score Requirement: 220
Minimum USMLE Step 2 Score Requirement: 220
Attempts on any step: Must pass on first attempt including CS exam
CS required at time of application: Yes including ECFMG certificate

USCE Requirement: None
Cut-Off time since graduation: 3 years
Program offers couple match: Yes
Visas Sponsored or accepted: J1 visa and H1b visa

St. Joseph Mercy-Oakland Transitional Year Residency Program

Specialty: Transitional Year
Program name: St Joseph Mercy-Oakland Program
Program code: 999-25-00-067
NRMP Code: 1319999P0
Program type: Community-based university affiliated hospital
State: Michigan
Address: St Joseph Mercy Oakland,
          44405 Woodward Ave, Pontiac, MI 48341
Phone: (248) 858-6233
Fax: (248) 858-3244
Percentage of IMGs in the program: 70%
Minimum USMLE Step 1 Score Requirement: 210
Minimum USMLE Step 2 Score Requirement: 210
Attempts on any step: Must pass on first attempt

CS required at time of application: No
USCE Requirement: None
Cut-Off time since graduation: 3 years
Program offers couple match: Yes
Visas Sponsored or accepted: J1 visa

Grand Rapids Medical Education Partners/Michigan State University Transitional Year Residency Program

Specialty: Transitional Year
Program name: Grand Rapids Medical Education Partners/Michigan State University Program
Program code: 999-25-00-190
NRMP Code: 2077999P0
Program type: Community-based
State: Michigan
Address: Grand Rapids Medical Education Partners,
            25 Michigan Ave NE, Grand Rapids, MI 49503
Phone: (616) 391-3245
Fax: (616) 391-3130
Percentage of IMGs in the program: 10%
Minimum USMLE Step 1 Score Requirement: No limits set

Minimum USMLE Step 2 Score Requirement:
No limits set
Attempts on any step: No limits set
CS required at time of application: No
USCE Requirement: Yes
Cut-Off time since graduation: 3 years
Program offers couple match: Yes
Visas Sponsored or accepted: J1 visa

Hurley Medical Center/Michigan State University Transitional Year Residency Program

Specialty: Transitional Year
Program name: Hurley Medical Center/Michigan State University Program
Program code: 999-25-00-062
NRMP Code: 1307999P1, 1307999P0
Program type: Community-based university affiliated hospital
State: Michigan
Address: Hurley Med Center,
          Two Hurley Plaza, Flint, MI 48503
Phone: (810) 262-9080
Fax: (810) 262-7245
Percentage of IMGs in the program: 50%
Minimum USMLE Step 1 Score Requirement:
213
Minimum USMLE Step 2 Score Requirement:
213

Attempts on any step: Maximum of 2 attempts on any step including CS exam
CS required at time of application: No
USCE Requirement: None
Cut-Off time since graduation: 5 years
Program offers couple match: Yes
Visas Sponsored or accepted: J1 visa and H1b visa

Detroit Medical Center/Wayne State University (Sinai-Grace) Transitional Year Residency Program

Specialty: Transitional Year
Program name: Detroit Medical Center/Wayne State University (Sinai-Grace) Program
Program code: 999-25-00-060
NRMP Code: 1374999P0, 1374999P1
Program type: University-based
State: Michigan
Address: Sinai-Grace Hospital,
6071 W Outer Dr, Detroit, MI 48235
Phone: (313) 966-3189
Fax: (313) 966-1738
Percentage of IMGs in the program: 80%
Minimum USMLE Step 1 Score Requirement: 200
Minimum USMLE Step 2 Score Requirement: 205

Attempts on any step: Must pass on first attempt
CS required at time of application: No
USCE Requirement: None
Cut-Off time since graduation: 3 years unless clinically active as in residency or practice
Program offers couple match: Yes
Visas Sponsored or accepted: J1 visa

Minnesota

Hennepin County Medical Center Transitional Year Residency Program

Specialty: Transitional Year
Program name: Hennepin County Medical Center Program
Program code: 999-26-00-069
 State: Minnesota
Address: Hennepin County Medical Center, 701 Park Ave S, Minneapolis, MN 55415-1829
Phone: (612) 873-3922
Fax: (612) 904-4401
Percentage of IMGs in the program: 10%

Minimum USMLE Step 1 Score Requirement: No limits set
Minimum USMLE Step 2 Score Requirement: No limits set
Attempts on any step: No limits set
CS required at time of application: No
USCE Requirement: None
Cut-Off time since graduation: No limits set
Program offers couple match: Yes
Visas Sponsored or accepted: No visa

New York

Lincoln Medical and Mental Health Center Transitional Year Residency Program

Specialty: Transitional Year
Program name: Lincoln Medical and Mental Health Center Program
Program code: 999-35-00-257
State: New York
Address: Lincoln Medical and Mental Health Center,
234 E 149th St, Bronx, NY 10451
Phone: (718) 579-5000
Fax: (718) 579-5246

Percentage of IMGs in the program: 30%
Minimum USMLE Step 1 Score Requirement: 210
Minimum USMLE Step 2 Score Requirement: 210
Attempts on any step: Must pass in first attempt
CS required at time of application: No
USCE Requirement: None
Cut-Off time since graduation: No limits set
Program offers couple match: Yes
Visas Sponsored or accepted: J1 visa and H1b visa

New York Medical College (Sound Shore) Transitional Year Residency Program

Specialty: Transitional Year
Program name: New York Medical College (Sound Shore) Program
Program code: 999-35-00-216
State: New York
Address: Sound Shore Medical Center Westchester,
        16 Guion Pl, New Rochelle, NY 10802
Phone: (914) 365-3681
Fax: (914) 365-5489

Percentage of IMGs in the program: 20%
Minimum USMLE Step 1 Score Requirement: 205
Minimum USMLE Step 2 Score Requirement: 205
Attempts on any step: Must pass on first attempt
CS required at time of application: No
USCE Requirement: None
Cut-Off time since graduation: 10 years
Program offers couple match: Yes
Visas Sponsored or accepted: J1 visa and H1b visa

United Health Services Hospitals Transitional Year Residency Program

Specialty: Transitional Year
Program name: United Health Services Hospitals Program
Program code: 999-35-00-081
NRMP Code: 1452999P0
Program type: Community-based university affiliated hospital
State: New York
Address: UHS Wilson Medical Center,
33-57 Harrison St, Johnson City, NY 13790
Phone: (800) 338-8471

Fax: (607) 798-1629
Percentage of IMGs in the program: 15%
Minimum USMLE Step 1 Score Requirement: 210
Minimum USMLE Step 2 Score Requirement: 210
Attempts on any step: No limits set
CS required at time of application: No
USCE Requirement: None
Cut-Off time since graduation: No limits set
Program offers couple match: Yes
Visas Sponsored or accepted: J1 visa and H1b visa

Ohio

Mount Carmel Health System Transitional Year Residency Program

Specialty: Transitional Year
Program name: Mount Carmel Health System Program
Program code: 999-38-00-093

State: Ohio
Address: Mount Carmel Health System,
            793 W State St, Columbus, OH 43222
Phone: (614) 234-1444 or (614) 234-1079
Fax: (614) 234-2772
Percentage of IMGs in the program: 25% (not every year they have IMGs)
Minimum USMLE Step 1 Score Requirement: 210
Minimum USMLE Step 2 Score Requirement: 210
Attempts on any step: Must pass on first attempt
CS required at time of application: Yes including ECFMG certificate
USCE Requirement: Yes
Cut-Off time since graduation: 5 years
Program offers couple match: Yes
Visas Sponsored or accepted: No visa

Pennsylvania

Mercy Catholic Medical Center Transitional Year Residency Program

Specialty: Transitional Year

Program name: Mercy Catholic Medical Center Program
Program code: 999-41-00-106
NRMP Code: 1636999P0
Program type: Community-based university affiliated hospital
State: Pennsylvania
Address: Mercy Catholic Medical Center,
           1500 Lansdowne Ave, Darby, PA 19023
Phone: (610) 237-4685
Fax: (610) 237-5093
Percentage of IMGs in the program: 35%
Minimum USMLE Step 1 Score Requirement: No limits set
Minimum USMLE Step 2 Score Requirement: No limits set
Attempts on any step: No limits set
CS required at time of application: No
USCE Requirement: No
Cut-Off time since graduation: No limits set
Program offers couple match: Yes
Visas Sponsored or accepted: J1 visa and H1b visa

UPMC Medical Education (Presbyterian Shadyside Hospital) Transitional Year Residency Program

Specialty: Transitional Year
Program name: UPMC Medical Education (Presbyterian Shadyside Hospital) Program
Program code: 999-41-00-117
State: Pennsylvania
Address: UPMC Presbyterian Shadyside, 5230 Centre Ave, Pittsburgh, PA 15232
Phone: (412) 623-2465
Fax: (412) 623-3592
Percentage of IMGs in the program: 35%
Minimum USMLE Step 1 Score Requirement: 204
Minimum USMLE Step 2 Score Requirement: 204
Attempts on any step: No limits set
CS required at time of application: Yes including ECFMG certificate
USCE Requirement: None
Cut-Off time since graduation: 2 years
Program offers couple match: Yes
Visas Sponsored or accepted: J1 visa and H1b visa

Wisconsin

Marshfield Clinic-St Joseph Hospital Transitional Year Residency Program

Specialty: Transitional Year
Program name: Marshfield Clinic-St Joseph's Hospital Program
Program code: 999-56-00-183
NRMP Code: 1780999P0
Program type: Community-based university affiliated hospital
State: Wisconsin
Address: Marshfield Clinic,
          1000 N Oak Ave, Marshfield, WI 54449
Phone: (715) 389-4151
Fax: (715) 389-4141
Percentage of IMGs in the program: 20%
Minimum USMLE Step 1 Score Requirement: 210
Minimum USMLE Step 2 Score Requirement: 210
Attempts on any step: No limits set
CS required at time of application: No
USCE Requirement: Yes
Cut-Off time since graduation: 3 years
Program offers couple match: Yes

Visas Sponsored or accepted: J1 visa and H1b visa

Table of Contents

Introduction 1

Connecticut 5

Yale-New Haven Hospital Transitional Year Residency Program 5

St. Vincent Medical Center Transitional Year Residency Program 6

Georgia 7

The Medical Center Transitional Year Residency Program 8

Emory University Transitional Year Residency Program...8

Illinois 9

Swedish Covenant Hospital Transitional Year Residency Program 10

Maryland 10

Maryland General Hospital Transitional Year Residency Program 11

Harbor Hospital Center Transitional Year Residency Program 12

Massachusetts 13

MetroWest Medical Center/Harvard Medical
School Transitional Year Residency Program
....13

Michigan..14

Oakwood Heritage Hospital Transitional Year
Residency Program 14

St. Mary Mercy Hospital Transitional Year
Residency Program 15

Wayne State University School of Medicine
Transitional Year Residency Program 16

Providence Hospital and Medical Centers
Transitional Year Residency Program 17

St. Joseph Mercy-Oakland Transitional Year
Residency Program 18

Grand Rapids Medical Education
Partners/Michigan State University
Transitional Year Residency Program 19

Hurley Medical Center/Michigan State
University Transitional Year Residency
Program...20

Detroit Medical Center/Wayne State
University (Sinai-Grace) Transitional Year
Residency Program 21

Minnesota 22

    Hennepin County Medical Center Transitional
    Year Residency Program 22

New York..23

    Lincoln Medical and Mental Health Center
    Transitional Year Residency Program 23

    New York Medical College (Sound Shore)
    Transitional Year Residency Program 24

    United Health Services Hospitals Transitional
    Year Residency Program 25

Ohio...26

    Mount Carmel Health System Transitional
    Year Residency Program 26

Pennsylvania 27

    Mercy Catholic Medical Center Transitional
    Year Residency Program 27

    UPMC Medical Education (Presbyterian
    Shadyside Hospital) Transitional Year
    Residency Program 29

Wisconsin..30

    Marshfield Clinic-St Joseph Hospital
    Transitional Year Residency Program 30

If you have any questions please email us at
applicantguide@yahoo.com

IMG Guide
&
Applicant Guide

www.imgguide.com
www.applicantguide.com

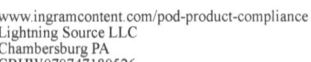